Home Remedies For Curing illness

A Guide to curing Sickness with Common Ingredients from Your home

Henry Steve

Table of content

Introduction

For centuries, people have turned to home remedies as a natural and affordable way to treat a variety of illnesses and ailments. These remedies often rely on ingredients that are readily available in the home or local environment, such as herbs, spices, fruits, and vegetables. While they may not be backed by scientific research, many people swear by the effectiveness of these remedies and continue to use them to this day.

Some of the most common home remedies include herbal teas, essential oils, honey, garlic, and ginger, all of which are believed to have powerful healing properties. These remedies can be used to treat everything from colds and flu to headaches, digestive issues, and skin problems.

While home remedies may not work for everyone and may not be appropriate for certain conditions, they can be a useful complement to conventional medical treatments. However, it's important to note that if you're experiencing severe symptoms or a medical emergency, you should always seek professional medical attention.

Definition of home remedies

Home remedies refer to natural or traditional remedies that are used to treat or alleviate common health problems or ailments using ingredients that are typically found in a household. These remedies are often passed down from generation to generation and may be based on cultural or traditional knowledge. Home remedies can include the use of herbs, spices, fruits, vegetables, oils, and other natural ingredients to promote healing and relieve symptoms. Some common examples of home remedies include using honey to soothe a sore throat, applying aloe Vera gel to sunburned skin, or drinking ginger tea to ease nausea. While home remedies may provide relief for certain health issues, it is important to consult with a healthcare provider before trying any new treatment.

Advantages of using home remedies

There are several advantages of using home remedies, including:

Cost-effective: Home remedies are often made from ingredients that are readily available in your kitchen or pantry, which makes them an affordable and cost-effective alternative to commercial products.

- **Natural:** Home remedies are often made from natural ingredients, which means they are free of synthetic chemicals that can be harmful to your health.
- **Easy to make:** Most home remedies are easy to make, and the recipes are readily available online or in books. You can make them at home without any special skills or equipment.

- **Safe:** Since home remedies are made from natural ingredients, they are generally considered safe for most people. However, it's important to note that some people may be allergic to certain ingredients, so it's always a good idea to test a small area first before using a new home remedy.

- **Potentially effective:** Home remedies have been used for centuries to treat various ailments, and many people find them to be effective. While scientific evidence may be limited for some remedies, many have been shown to have potential benefits.

- **Personalized:** Home remedies can be customized to suit your specific needs and preferences. For example, you can adjust the concentration of ingredients or add other ingredients to a recipe to make it more effective or palatable.

Overall, home remedies can be a convenient, cost-effective, and safe option for treating minor health issues or promoting overall wellness.

Importance of knowing about home remedies

Knowing about home remedies can be important for several reasons:

- **Accessibility:** Home remedies are often made from ingredients that are readily available in your home or at a local store, making them more accessible than prescription medications or expensive treatments.

- **Affordability:** Home remedies are often less expensive than prescription medications or medical treatments, making them a more affordable option for people who may not have access to healthcare or who cannot afford expensive treatments.

- **Convenience:** Home remedies can be administered at home, without the need for a doctor's appointment or a trip to the pharmacy. This can be especially important for people who live in remote areas or who have limited mobility.

- **Safety:** Home remedies are often made from natural ingredients, which can be safer and have fewer side effects than prescription medications. However, it is important to note that not all home remedies are safe or effective, and some can even be harmful.

- **Empowerment:** Knowing about home remedies can empower people to take control of their health and wellbeing, and to try natural remedies before resorting to more invasive or expensive treatments.

Overall, while home remedies may not always be a substitute for medical care, they can be a useful tool for managing minor ailments or symptoms, and for promoting overall health and wellbeing.

Chapter 1:

common ailments and their home remedies

Cold and flu

These are respiratory illnesses caused by viruses. The common cold is caused by rhinoviruses, while influenza (flu) is caused by the influenza virus.

The symptoms of cold and flu can include:

- Runny or stuffy nose
- Sore throat
- Cough
- Congestion
- Body aches
- Fatigue
- Fever

Some home remedies include:

- **Stay hydrated:** Drinking plenty of fluids, such as water, tea, or soup, can help loosen mucus and keep you hydrated.
- **Rest:** Getting plenty of rest can help your body fight off the virus and speed up your recovery.
- **Gargle salt water:** Gargling with warm salt water can help soothe a sore throat and reduce inflammation.

- **Steam:** Inhaling steam from a hot shower or a bowl of hot water with a towel over your head can help relieve congestion.
- **Use a humidifier:** Keeping the air moist with a humidifier can help ease congestion and soothe a sore throat.
- **Honey:** Adding honey to hot tea or warm water can help soothe a cough and sore throat.
- **Vitamin C:** Consuming foods high in vitamin C, such as oranges, lemons, and kiwi, can help boost your immune system and potentially reduce the duration of your illness.

Sore throat

A sore throat is a common condition that can cause discomfort or pain in the throat. It can be caused by a variety of factors, including viral or bacterial infections, allergies, dry air, or acid reflux.

Some home remedies for a sore throat include:

- **Gargling with warm salt water:** Mix a half teaspoon of salt into a glass of warm water and gargle it for 30 seconds before spitting it out. This can help reduce both the inflammation pain.
- **Drinking warm liquids:** Sipping warm liquids such as tea, broth or soup can help soothe a sore throat.
- **Using throat lozenges:** Throat lozenges can provide temporary relief by numbing the throat or providing a coating that protects it from further irritation.

- **Resting your voice:** Speaking too much or too loudly can exacerbate a sore throat, so it's important to rest your voice as much as possible.

- **Humidifying the air:** A humidifier can add moisture to the air and alleviate dryness that can contribute to a sore throat.

- **Over-the-counter pain relief:** Pain relievers such as acetaminophen or ibuprofen can help reduce pain and fever associated with a sore throat.

- **Honey and lemon:** Mixing honey and lemon in warm water and sipping it can help soothe a sore throat. Honey has antibacterial properties while lemon has vitamin C, which can boost the immune system.

- **Garlic:** Garlic has antibacterial and antiviral properties that can help fight infections. Chewing a raw garlic clove or adding it to food can help relieve a sore throat.

- **Apple cider vinegar:** Gargling with a mixture of apple cider vinegar and warm water can help kill bacteria and relieve pain.

Headaches

these are a common condition characterized by pain or discomfort in the head or neck region. They can be caused by a variety of factors, such as stress, tension, dehydration, lack of sleep, eyestrain, or certain medical conditions.

some home remedies include:

- **Stay hydrated:** Drinking plenty of water can help prevent dehydration, which can trigger headaches.

- **Apply a cold compress:** Placing a cold compress, such as a bag of frozen peas, on your forehead or neck can help reduce pain and inflammation.

- **Take a warm bath:** Soaking in a warm bath or using a warm towel on your neck or shoulders can help relax tense muscles that may be causing the headache.
- **Get enough rest:** Getting enough sleep and taking breaks throughout the day can help reduce stress and prevent tension headaches.
- **Practice relaxation techniques:** Techniques such as deep breathing, meditation, or yoga can help reduce stress and tension that may contribute to headaches.
- **Use essential oils:** Peppermint, lavender, and eucalyptus essential oils may help alleviate headaches when applied topically or inhaled.
- **Avoid triggers:** Identify and avoid any triggers that may be causing your headaches, such as certain foods, caffeine, or bright lights.

Indigestion

This is also known as dyspepsia, it is a common digestive problem that occurs when your stomach acid comes in contact with the lining of your digestive system, causing discomfort and pain. Some of the symptoms of indigestion include bloating, nausea, heartburn, and stomach pain.

some home remedies for indigestion:

- **Ginger:** Ginger is known for its ability to reduce inflammation in the digestive system. You can take ginger in the form of ginger tea, ginger ale, or simply chew on a piece of raw ginger.

- **Baking soda:** Baking soda can neutralize the excess stomach acid that causes indigestion. Mix a teaspoon of baking soda with a glass of water and drink it slowly.
- **Apple cider vinegar:** Apple cider vinegar helps to reduce the acidity in your stomach. Mix one tablespoon of apple cider vinegar with a glass of water and drink it slowly.
- **Fennel seeds:** Fennel seeds contain anethole, a compound that can help to relax the stomach muscles and reduce bloating. You can chew on fennel seeds or make tea by boiling them in water.
- **Peppermint:** Peppermint can help to soothe the digestive system and reduce nausea. You can drink peppermint tea or chew on a peppermint leaf.
- **Chamomile tea:** Chamomile tea can help to reduce inflammation in the digestive system and calm the stomach. Drink chamomile tea after meals to help prevent indigestion.
- **Avoid trigger foods:** Certain foods like fatty or spicy foods, caffeine, alcohol, and carbonated drinks can trigger indigestion. Avoid these foods if you are prone to indigestion.

Constipation

this is a condition in which an individual experiences difficulty in passing stools or has infrequent bowel movements. It is generally characterized by hard, dry, and small stools that are difficult to pass.

Some home remedies include:

- **Increase your water intake:** Drinking more water can help soften your stools and make them easier to pass.
- **Eat more fiber:** Fiber can help add bulk to your stools and make them easier to pass. Great sources of fiber include fruits, vegetables, whole grains, and legumes.
- **Exercise regularly:** Physical activity can help stimulate the muscles in your digestive system, making it easier to pass stools.
- **Drink warm liquids:** Drinking warm liquids, such as herbal tea or warm water with lemon, can help stimulate your digestive system and relieve constipation.
- **Try natural laxatives:** Certain foods, such as prunes, figs, and kiwi, have natural laxative properties that can help relieve constipation.
- **Massage your abdomen:** Massaging your abdomen in a circular motion can help stimulate your digestive system and relieve constipation.
- **Use the bathroom when you feel the urge:** Ignoring the urge to have a bowel movement can make constipation worse

Diarrhea

This is a condition characterized by loose, watery stools occurring more than three times a day. It can be caused by a variety of factors, including viral or bacterial infections, food allergies or intolerances, certain medications, and medical conditions like inflammatory bowel disease.

some home remedies for diarrhea include:

- **Stay hydrated:** Drink plenty of fluids like water, coconut water, clear broths, or electrolyte drinks to prevent dehydration.

- **Consume probiotics:** Yogurt or other foods containing live and active cultures can help replenish the good bacteria in your gut.

- **Eat bland foods:** Stick to easily digestible, low-fiber foods like bananas, rice, applesauce, and toast (BRAT diet).

- **Avoid certain foods:** Avoid dairy, caffeine, alcohol, and greasy or spicy foods until your symptoms improve.

- **Take over-the-counter medications:** Anti-diarrheal medications like loperamide or bismuth subsalicylate can help slow down bowel movements and relieve symptoms.

- **Rest:** Resting can help your body recover and reduce stress on your digestive system.

Insomnia

this is a sleep disorder characterized by difficulty falling asleep or staying asleep, or waking up too early and not being able to go back to sleep. It can cause fatigue, daytime sleepiness, irritability, and difficulty concentrating.

Some home remedies for insomnia include:

- **Stick to a sleep schedule:** Going to bed and waking up at the same time every day can help regulate your body's sleep-wake cycle.

- **Create a relaxing bedtime routine:** Activities such as reading a book, taking a warm bath, or listening to soothing music can help you wind down and prepare for sleep.

- **Avoid both caffeine and alcohol:** Both caffeine and alcohol can interfere with sleep. It's best to avoid them altogether or limit your intake, especially in the evening.

- **Exercise regularly:** Regular physical activity can help improve sleep quality, but it's important to exercise earlier in the day as exercise close to bedtime may actually make it harder to fall asleep.

- **Avoid daytime napping:** If you have trouble sleeping at night, it's best to avoid napping during the day.

- **Create a sleep-conducive environment:** Make sure your bedroom is cool, quiet, and dark, and consider using comfortable bedding and pillows.

- **Consider relaxation techniques:** Techniques such as deep breathing, progressive muscle relaxation, and meditation may help you relax and fall asleep.

natural remedies for skin problems

Acne

This is a common skin condition that occurs when hair follicles become clogged with oil and dead skin cells. The resulting inflammation can lead to pimples, blackheads, and whiteheads, as well as more severe forms of acne such as nodules and cysts.

Some natural remedies for acne include:

- **Tea tree oil:** This essential oil has antimicrobial properties that can help kill the bacteria that contribute to acne.
- **Aloe Vera:** Aloe Vera gel can help soothe inflammation and redness associated with acne.
- **Apple cider vinegar:** This vinegar can help balance the pH of the skin, which can reduce the risk of acne.
- **Honey:** Honey has antibacterial properties that can help fight acne-causing bacteria.
- **Green tea:** Drinking green tea or using it topically can help reduce inflammation and improve the appearance of acne-prone skin.
- **Zinc:** Taking zinc supplements or using topical zinc can help reduce inflammation and improve the healing of acne.
- **Witch hazel:** This natural astringent can help reduce oil production and soothe irritated skin.

Eczema

This is also known as atopic dermatitis, is a common skin condition that causes redness, dryness, and itchiness. It can occur anywhere on the body, but it typically appears on the face, hands, feet, and folds of the skin. Eczema is often caused by a combination of genetic and environmental factors, such as allergies or stress.

Some natural remedies for eczema, include:

- **Coconut oil:** Coconut oil has anti-inflammatory and moisturizing properties that can help soothe and hydrate the skin. Apply a thin layer of coconut oil to the affected areas after bathing or showering.
- **Oatmeal baths:** Oatmeal contains compounds that can help reduce inflammation and itchiness. Add a cup of colloidal oatmeal to your bathwater and soak for 10-15 minutes.
- **Aloe Vera:** Aloe Vera contains compounds that can help reduce inflammation and promote healing. Apply aloe Vera gel on the areas affected several times a day.
- **Chamomile tea:** Chamomile has anti-inflammatory properties that can help soothe and calm the skin. Brew a strong chamomile tea, let it cool, and apply it to the affected areas with a cotton ball.
- **Probiotics:** Probiotics can help improve gut health and boost the immune system, which may help reduce eczema symptoms. Eat foods that are rich in probiotics, such as yogurt, kefir, and sauerkraut, or take a probiotic supplement.

this is a chronic autoimmune condition that causes skin cells to build up rapidly, leading to scaly, itchy, and inflamed patches of skin. These patches can appear on any part of the body, but are most commonly found on the elbows, knees, scalp, and lower back.

Some natural remedies for psoriasis include:

- **Aloe Vera:** The gel from the aloe Vera plant can soothe and moisturize inflamed skin. Apply it directly to the affected area.
- **Oatmeal baths:** Adding colloidal oatmeal to a warm bath can help relieve itching and inflammation.
- **Turmeric:** Turmeric has anti-inflammatory properties and can help reduce psoriasis symptoms. You can add it to your food or take it as a supplement.
- **Tea tree oil:** Tea tree oil has antimicrobial properties and can help reduce inflammation. Dilute it with a carrier oil and apply it to the area affected.
- **Omega-3 fatty acids:** Omega-3 fatty acids can help reduce inflammation and may improve psoriasis symptoms. You can get them from fatty fish, such as salmon, or take a supplement.

Sunburn

this is a type of skin damage that occurs due to overexposure to the ultraviolet (UV) radiation of the sun. The symptoms of sunburn include redness, pain, swelling, blistering, and peeling of the affected skin.

Some natural remedies for sunburn include:

- **Aloe Vera:** Aloe Vera has anti-inflammatory properties and can help soothe sunburned skin. Just apply aloe Vera gel directly to the area affected.
- **Cool compress:** Applying a cool compress, such as a damp towel or cloth, to the sunburned area can help reduce inflammation and provide relief.
- **Apple Cider Vinegar:** Diluted apple cider vinegar can help reduce pain and inflammation associated with sunburn. Mix equal parts of water and apple cider vinegar and apply to the affected area using a cotton ball.
- **Coconut oil:** Coconut oil has moisturizing properties that can help reduce peeling and promote healing. Apply a thin layer of coconut oil to the area affected.
- **Oatmeal:** Oatmeal has anti-inflammatory properties that can help soothe sunburned skin. Add a cup of oatmeal to a bathtub of lukewarm water and soak for 15-20 minutes.

Dry skin

This is a common skin condition characterized by flaky, itchy, or rough patches of skin that may feel tight or uncomfortable. It occurs when the skin lacks sufficient moisture or natural oils, causing it to lose its elasticity and become prone to cracking and irritation.

Some natural remedies for dry skin include:

- **Drink plenty of water:** Staying hydrated is essential for maintaining healthy skin. Drinking at least 8-10 glasses of water a day can help to keep your skin moisturized from the inside out.

- **Use a humidifier:** Dry air can exacerbate dry skin. Using a humidifier can help to add moisture to the air, which can prevent your skin from becoming too dry.

- **Apply natural oils:** Coconut oil, almond oil, and olive oil are all great options for moisturizing dry skin. Just apply a little amount to the affected area and massage gently until it's absorbed fully.

- **Oatmeal baths:** Oatmeal contains natural anti-inflammatory properties and can help to soothe itchy, dry skin. Add a cup of oatmeal to your bathwater and soak for 10-15 minutes.

- **Avoid hot showers:** Hot water can strip your skin of its natural oils, exacerbating dryness. Stick to lukewarm water when showering or bathing, and avoid spending too much time in the water.

- **Use gentle, natural cleansers:** Harsh soaps and cleansers can strip your skin of its natural oils, causing it to become dry and irritated. Opt for gentle, natural cleansers that are free from harsh chemicals and fragrances.

Chapter 3:

Home Remedies for Pain Relief

Back pain

This refers to discomfort or pain felt anywhere along the spine, from the neck to the hips. It can range from a dull ache to a sharp stabbing sensation, and may be caused by a variety of factors, including poor posture, muscle strain, injury, or underlying medical conditions.

Some home remedies for back pain include:

- **Heat therapy:** Applying a heating pad or taking a warm bath or shower can help relax tense muscles and improve blood flow to the affected area.
- **Cold therapy**: Applying a cold pack or ice wrapped in a towel to the affected area can help reduce inflammation and numb the pain.
- **Stretching:** Gentle stretching exercises can help loosen tight muscles and improve flexibility.
- **Exercise:** Regular physical activity can help strengthen the muscles in your back and improve your overall posture.
- **Massage:** Massaging the affected area can help relax tense muscles and improve circulation.
- **Yoga or Pilates:** These exercises can help improve flexibility and strengthen the muscles in your back and core.
- **Over-the-counter pain relievers:** Medications such as ibuprofen or acetaminophen can help alleviate pain and reduce inflammation.

This refers to pain that originates from a tooth or its surrounding area, which can be caused by a variety of factors such as tooth decay, gum disease, dental abscess, tooth fracture or injury, and teeth grinding.

Some home remedies for toothache include:

- **Saltwater rinse:** Mix a teaspoon of salt in a cup of warm water, and rinse your mouth with it for 30 seconds before spitting it out. Repeat several times a day to reduce inflammation and fight bacteria.
- **Clove oil:** Apply a small amount of clove oil on the affected tooth or gum using a cotton ball. Clove oil contains eugenol, a natural analgesic and antibacterial agent that can numb the pain and reduce inflammation.
- **Garlic:** Crush a garlic clove and mix it with a pinch of salt, then apply it to the affected tooth. Garlic contains allicin, a natural antibiotic that can kill bacteria and relieve pain.
- **Peppermint tea bags:** Steep a peppermint tea bag in hot water, then let it cool down and place it on the affected tooth or gum. Peppermint has a cooling and numbing effect that can provide temporary relief from pain.
- **Hydrogen peroxide:** Mix equal parts of hydrogen peroxide and water, and swish it In your mouth for 30 seconds before spitting it out. Hydrogen peroxide kills bacteria and reduce inflammation.

Joint pain

This is a common problem that can affect people of all ages. It is characterized by pain, discomfort, or inflammation in one or more of the joints in the body, such as the knees, hips, wrists, shoulders, or ankles. There are several factors that can contribute to joint pain, including injury, arthritis, overuse, or autoimmune diseases.

Some natural remedies for joint pain include:

- **Exercise:** Regular exercise can help strengthen the muscles around the joints, improve flexibility, and reduce joint pain. Low-impact exercises like swimming, yoga, or walking can be particularly beneficial for people with joint pain.

- **Hot and cold therapy:** Applying heat or cold to the area affected can help reduce pain and inflammation. A warm compress or heating pad can help relax the muscles and increase blood flow to the joint, while a cold compress or ice pack can help numb the area and reduce swelling.

- **Massage:** Gentle massage can help relieve tension and improve circulation around the joint. Using essential oils like peppermint or lavender oil during the massage can also provide additional pain relief.

- **Turmeric:** this is a natural anti-inflammatory agent that can help reduce joint pain and stiffness. Adding turmeric to your diet or taking turmeric supplements can be an effective way to alleviate joint pain.

- **Omega-3 fatty acids:** Omega-3 fatty acids found in fish oil can help reduce inflammation and joint pain. Eating fatty fish like salmon, mackerel, or tuna, or taking fish oil supplements, can be an effective way to incorporate omega-3s into your diet.

Muscle pain

This is also known as myalgia, is a common condition that can be caused by a variety of factors such as tension, overuse, injury, or certain medical conditions. It can be a dull ache or a sharp, stabbing pain and can affect any muscle in the body.

Some home remedies for muscle pain include:

- **Rest:** Avoid activities that may cause further strain to the affected muscle and take time to rest and recover.
- **Apply Heat or Cold:** Applying heat or cold to the affected area can help reduce inflammation and pain. Use a hot compress or heating pad for 15-20 minutes at a time, or a cold compress or ice pack for 10-15 minutes at a time.
- **Massage:** Gently massaging the affected area can help improve blood circulation and reduce muscle tension. Use gentle circular motions with your fingers or a massage ball.
- **Stretching:** Gentle stretching can help relieve muscle pain and tension. Try to stretch the affected muscle slowly and hold the stretch for 15-30 seconds.
- **Drink Plenty of Water:** Dehydration can exacerbate muscle pain, so it's important to drink plenty of water to stay hydrated.
- **Take a Warm Bath:** Soaking in a warm bath with Epsom salt can help relax the muscles and reduce pain.
- **Get Enough Sleep:** Make sure you're getting enough restful sleep to allow your muscles to recover and heal.

Chapter 4:

Alternative Remedies for Mental Health

Anxiety

This is a normal human emotion that is characterized by feelings of worry, fear, or unease about uncertain outcomes or potential threats. However, when anxiety becomes excessive and interferes with daily activities, it may be considered an anxiety disorder.

Some common symptoms of anxiety include; excessive worry, restlessness, irritability, difficulty concentrating, muscle tension, and sleep disturbances.

Some alternative remedies for anxiety include:

- **Mindfulness and relaxation techniques:** Techniques such as deep breathing, meditation, yoga, and progressive muscle relaxation can help reduce stress and anxiety.
- **Exercise:** Regular exercise has been shown to be an effective way to reduce anxiety symptoms.
- **A healthy diet:** A balanced diet that includes whole grains, fruits, vegetables, lean proteins, and healthy fats may help reduce anxiety.
- **Supplements:** Some natural supplements, such as magnesium, chamomile, and valerian root, may help reduce anxiety symptoms.

- **Therapy:** Cognitive-behavioral therapy (CBT) is a type of talk therapy that can help individuals learn to manage their anxiety by changing negative thought patterns and behaviors.

Depression

This is a mental health condition characterized by persistent feelings of sadness, hopelessness, and a loss of interest in daily activities. It can affect a person's ability to function normally and may interfere with their relationships, work, and daily life. Depression is usually caused by a combination of genetic, environmental, and psychological factors.

There are many different treatments for depression, including:

- **Psychotherapy:** This type of therapy involves talking with a mental health professional to identify and address the underlying causes of depression. Different forms of therapy, such as cognitive-behavioral therapy, can help individuals change negative thought patterns and behaviors that contribute to depression.
- **Medications:** Antidepressants are commonly prescribed to treat depression. They work by altering the levels of certain chemicals in the brain, such as serotonin and norepinephrine, which can improve mood and reduce symptoms.
- **Exercise:** Regular physical activity has been shown to be an effective way to manage depression. Exercise can increase endorphins, reduce stress, and improve sleep, all of which can help alleviate symptoms of depression.

- **Mindfulness meditation:** This involves paying attention to the present moment without judgment. Mindfulness meditation can help individuals become more aware of their thoughts and feelings, and can help reduce symptoms of depression.

- **Nutritional supplements:** Certain supplements, such as omega-3 fatty acids and vitamin D, have been shown to improve symptoms of depression. However, it's important to speak with a healthcare provider before taking any supplements, as they may interact with other medications.

- **Light therapy:** For individuals with seasonal affective disorder (SAD), a type of depression that occurs during the winter months, light therapy may be effective. Light therapy involves exposure to bright light for a set period of time each day.

Stress

This is a psychological and physiological response to a perceived threat or demand. It can be caused by various factors such as work pressure, relationship issues, financial problems, health concerns, and more. Stress can have negative effects on both mental and physical health, including anxiety, depression, insomnia, high blood pressure, and heart disease.

Some alternative remedies for stress include:

- **Exercise:** Regular exercise has been shown to reduce stress levels by releasing endorphins, improving mood, and reducing tension in the body.

- **Meditation and Mindfulness:** Mindfulness meditation practices can help reduce stress and improve overall mental wellbeing. It involves focusing on the present moment, without judgment or distraction, and allowing thoughts and emotions to pass without attachment.

- **Yoga:** Practicing yoga can help reduce stress by combining physical postures, breathing techniques, and meditation practices.
- **Deep Breathing:** Deep breathing exercises can help reduce stress and anxiety by slowing down the heart rate, lowering blood pressure, and relaxing the body.
- **Social Support:** Talking to a friend or family member can help reduce stress by providing emotional support and a sense of belonging.
- **Time Management:** Learning to prioritize tasks and manage time effectively can help reduce stress levels by preventing overload and overwhelm.
- **Herbal Remedies:** Some herbs such as chamomile, lavender, and passionflower have been shown to have calming effects on the body and may help reduce stress levels.
- **Get Enough Sleep:** Make sure you're getting enough restful sleep to allow your muscles to recover and heal.

Chapter 5:

Remedies for Common Household Injuries

Cuts and bruises

These are two types of injuries that can occur as a result of physical trauma.

Cuts occur when the skin is broken or lacerated, often due to a sharp object such as a knife or broken glass. Bruises, on the other hand, occur when the body experiences blunt force trauma, such as a fall or a blow.

Some home remedies for cuts and bruises include:

- **Clean the wound:** For cuts, clean the wound thoroughly with soap and water. Dry the affected area with a clean towel. This helps to prevent infection.
- **Apply pressure:** To stop bleeding from a cut, apply pressure to the wound with a clean cloth or bandage.
- **Use ice:** For bruises, apply an ice pack to the affected area for 20-30 minutes at a time, several times a day. This will help to reduce the swelling and pain.
- **Elevate the affected area:** For bruises on the arms or legs, elevate the affected limb above heart level. This helps to reduce swelling.
- **Apply arnica cream:** Arnica cream, derived from a plant, can help to reduce swelling and bruising. Apply it to the area affected several times a day.

- **Apply honey:** Honey has antibacterial properties and can help to prevent infection in cuts. Apply a small amount of honey to the wound and cover with a bandage.
- **Drink water:** Drinking plenty of water can help to flush toxins out of the body, which can aid in the healing process.

Burns

This refers to skin injuries that occur due to heat, radiation, electricity, or chemicals. The severity of the burn depends on the depth and extent of the injury.

Some home remedies for healing minor burns include:

- **Cool water:** Hold the affected area under cool (not cold) running water for 10 to 15 mlnutes or apply a cold, damp compress. This can help to reduce swelling, ease pain, and prevent further tissue damage.
- **Aloe Vera:** Apply a thin layer of aloe Vera gel or aloe Vera cream to the burn. Aloe Vera has anti-inflammatory properties that can help soothe the skin and promote healing.
- **Honey:** Apply a thin layer of honey to the burn and cover with a sterile dressing. Honey has antimicrobial properties that can help prevent infection and promote healing.
- **Tea bags:** Soak a tea bag in cool water and apply it to the burn. The tannic acid in tea can help to soothe the skin and reduce pain.
- **Coconut oll:** Apply a thin layer of coconut oil to the burn. Coconut oil has anti-inflammatory properties that can help soothe the skin and promote healing.

Insect bites and stings

These occur when an insect, such as a mosquito, bee, wasp, or ant, injects its venom or saliva into your skin. This can cause a range of symptoms, from mild irritation to severe allergic reactions.

Some common home remedies for insect bites and stings include:

- **Apply a cold compress:** This can help reduce swelling and pain. You can use a cold pack on the area affected or wrap some ice in a towel and put on it.
- **Take an antihistamine:** This can help reduce itching and swelling. You can take an over-the-counter antihistamine such as Benadryl.
- **Apply calamine lotion:** This can help soothe the itchiness and provide some relief.
- **Use baking soda:** Mix baking soda with water to create a paste and apply it to the bite or sting. This can help neutralize the venom and reduce itching.
- **Apply apple cider vinegar:** Soak a cotton ball in apple cider vinegar and apply it to the bite or sting. This can help reduce itching and swelling.
- **Use essential oils:** Certain essential oils, such as tea tree oil or lavender oil, have anti-inflammatory and soothing properties that can help relieve the symptoms of insect bites and stings.

Chapter 6:

Remedies for Children

Fever

this is a common symptom in children that usually indicates an infection or illness. It is defined as a temperature of 100.4 degrees Fahrenheit (38 degrees Celsius) or higher, taken orally. While fever itself is not usually harmful, it can make your child feel uncomfortable and irritable.

Here are some home remedies that can help manage your child's fever:

- **Keep your child hydrated:** Encourage your child to drink plenty of fluids, such as water, clear broths, and electrolyte solutions to prevent dehydration.
- **Dress your child appropriately:** Dress your child in lightweight, breathable clothing and cover them with a light blanket if they feel cold.
- **Give a lukewarm bath:** A lukewarm bath can help reduce your child's body temperature. Avoid using cold water or alcohol rubs, as they can cause shivering and increase the body temperature.
- **Use fever-reducing medication:** Over the counter fever-reducing medications like acetaminophen and ibuprofen can help reduce fever and relieve discomfort. Follow the dosing instructions carefully and consult your child's healthcare provider if you have any questions.
- **Provide a cool and comfortable environment:** Keep your child's room cool and well-ventilated, and use a fan to circulate the air.

Colds and coughs

These are common respiratory infections that affect children of all ages. Colds are caused by viruses that infect the upper respiratory tract, including the nose, throat, and sinuses. Symptoms of a cold include runny nose, nasal congestion, sneezing, sore throat, cough, and sometimes fever.

Coughs, on the other hand, can be caused by a variety of factors such as viral or bacterial infections, allergies, asthma, or exposure to irritants. A cough can be either dry or productive (with phlegm).

Here are some home remedies for children's colds and coughs:

- **Honey:** Honey is a natural cough suppressant that can soothe irritated throat. It can be given to children above one year of age. Mix 1-2 teaspoons of honey in a glass of warm water and give it to your child before bedtime.
- **Steam inhalation:** Inhaling steam can help clear the nasal passages and relieve congestion. You can run a hot shower or use a humidifier in your child's room.
- **Saline drops:** Saline drops can be used to clear the nasal passages in babies and young children. You can use a dropper to apply a few drops in each nostril.
- **Rest:** Rest is important for your child's recovery. Ensure your child rest and avoid strenuous activities.
- **Fluids:** It is important to keep your child hydrated when they have a cold or cough. Encourage them to drink plenty of fluids like water, fruit juice, or warm broth.

- **Vitamin C:** Foods rich in vitamin C, such as citrus fruits, can help boost your child's immune system and reduce the severity of cold symptoms.

Earaches

These are a common problem in children and can be caused by a variety of reasons, including ear infections, wax buildup, sinus infections, or allergies.

Here are some home remedies for pain and discomfort associated with earaches in children:

- **Warm compress:** A warm compress can help ease the pain of an earache. Soak a washcloth in warm water, wring out the excess water, and place it over the affected ear.
- **Olive oil:** Warm a few drops of olive oil and use a dropper to put them in the affected ear. This can help to loosen any wax buildup that may be causing the pain.
- **Garlic oil:** Garlic has natural antibacterial properties that can help fight off infection. Crush a clove of garlic and mix it with a few drops of olive oil. Warm the mixture and use a dropper to put a few drops in the affected ear.
- **Hydrogen peroxide:** Mix equal parts of hydrogen peroxide and water and use a dropper to put a few drops in the affected ear. This can help to remove any wax buildup that may be causing the pain.
- **Elevate the head:** If your child is lying down, prop their head up with a pillow. This can help to ease the pressure in the ear.

This refers to the discomfort or pain experienced by infants and young children as their first set of teeth emerge through their gums. The teething process typically starts at around 6 months of age and can continue until the child is about 3 years old.

The symptoms of teething can vary from child to child, but some common signs include; drooling, swollen or tender gums, irritability, restlessness, loss of appetite, and disturbed sleep.

Here are some home remedies that can help alleviate teething pain in children:

- **Cold objects:** Giving your child something cold to chew on, such as a chilled teething ring, a cold washcloth, or a frozen piece of banana, can help numb the gums and provide relief.
- **Pressure:** Gently massaging your child's gums with a clean finger or a soft, wet cloth can also help alleviate teething pain.
- **Pain-relieving gels:** Over-the-counter pain-relieving gels, such as those containing benzocaine or lidocaine, can be applied directly to your child's gums to help numb the pain. However, it's important to follow the instructions carefully and not use these gels excessively.
- **Acetaminophen or ibuprofen:** If your child is experiencing severe teething pain, you can give them a pain reliever such as acetaminophen or ibuprofen, but only after consulting with their pediatrician and following the recommended dosage.
- **Distraction:** Engaging your child in play or offering them a favorite toy or book can help take their mind off the discomfort of teething.

- **Breastfeeding or bottle feeding:** For infants, nursing or bottle feeding can provide comfort and help alleviate teething pain.

Stomach pain

This is also known as abdominal pain, is a common condition in children. It can be caused by a variety of factors, including constipation, indigestion, gas, food allergies, and infections. The pain can range from mild to severe and can be accompanied by other symptoms such as nausea, vomiting, and diarrhea.

Here are some home remedies that can help alleviate stomach pain in children:

- **Encourage rest:** Rest is important for the body to recover from any discomfort or pain. Encourage your child to rest in a comfortable position and avoid strenuous activities.

- **Provide plenty of fluids:** Offer your child plenty of fluids such as water, clear broths, or electrolyte solutions like Pedialyte. This can help prevent dehydration and ease constipation.

- **Use heat:** Applying a warm compress or heating pad to the stomach can help soothe the pain. Just make sure it's not too hot and avoid leaving it on for too long.

- **Offer a bland diet:** Avoid spicy, fatty, or fried foods that can aggravate the stomach. Instead, offer a bland diet such as bananas, rice, applesauce, and toast.

- **Try herbal tea:** Chamomile, peppermint, and ginger teas can help ease stomach pain and nausea. Just make sure to offer them in moderation and avoid any teas with caffeine.

- **Consult with a healthcare provider:** If your child's stomach pain persists or worsens, it's important to seek medical advice from a healthcare provider.

Chapter 7:

Remedies for Women's Health

Menstrual cramps

This is also known as dysmenorrhea, are painful sensations that occur before or during menstruation. These cramps are caused by the uterus contracting to help shed its lining. The pain can increase from mild to severe and can last for a few hours to even a few days.

Some remedies for menstrual cramps include:

- **Over-the-counter pain relievers:** Nonsteroidal anti-inflammatory drugs (NSAIDs) such as Ibuprofen, naproxen, and aspirin can help reduce menstrual cramp pain.

- **Heat therapy:** Applying a heating pad or taking a warm bath or shower can help relax the muscles and reduce pain.

- **Exercise:** Light exercise such as yoga, walking, or stretching can help relieve menstrual cramps by increasing blood flow and reducing stress.

- **Dietary changes:** Eating a healthy, balanced diet that is rich in fruits, vegetables, and whole grains can help reduce menstrual cramps.

- **Herbal remedies:** Some herbs, such as ginger, cinnamon, and chamomile, may help reduce menstrual cramps.

A yeast infection, also known as candidiasis, is a fungal infection caused by an overgrowth of yeast in the body, usually in warm and moist areas such as the mouth, vagina, or skin folds.

Common symptoms of a yeast infection include; itching, burning, and redness in the affected area, as well as white discharge (in the case of vaginal yeast infections).

There are several remedies for yeast infections, including:

- **Over-the-counter antifungal medications:** These are creams, ointments, or suppositories that can be purchased at a pharmacy without a prescription.
- **Prescription antifungal medications:** If the over-the-counter treatments are not effective, a doctor may prescribe a stronger medication.
- **Probiotics:** Eating foods that contain live cultures, such as yogurt or taking probiotic supplements, may help prevent yeast infections by promoting a healthy balance of bacteria in the body.
- **Avoiding certain foods:** Yeast feeds on sugar, so avoiding sugary and processed foods may help prevent the overgrowth of yeast.
- **Keeping the affected area clean and dry:** This can help prevent the growth of yeast and may help reduce symptoms.

UTI

This stands for urinary tract infection, which is a common infection that occurs in the urinary system, which includes the bladder, kidneys, ureters, and urethra.

The symptoms of a UTI can include; a strong and frequent urge to urinate, a burning sensation during urination, cloudy or foul-smelling urine, and pain in the lower abdomen or back.

Here are some remedies that may help to relieve the symptoms of a UTI:

- **Drink plenty of water:** Staying hydrated can help to flush bacteria out of the urinary tract.
- **Take over-the-counter pain medication:** Nonsteroidal anti-inflammatory drugs (NSAIDs) such as ibuprofen can help to relieve pain and reduce inflammation.
- **Use a heating pad:** Placing a heating pad on your lower abdomen can help to relieve pain and discomfort.
- **Take probiotics:** Consuming probiotic-rich foods or taking probiotic supplements may help to restore healthy bacteria in the urinary tract.
- **Avoid irritants:** Avoiding irritants such as caffeine, alcohol, and spicy foods may help to reduce symptoms.
- **Antibiotics:** Antibiotics are typically the primary treatment for UTIs. If your symptoms persist or worsen, it is important to see a doctor to get a prescription for antibiotics.

Chapter 8:

Precautions and Safety Measures

Guidelines for safe use of home remedies

While home remedies can be effective and convenient, it is important to use them safely to avoid any potential risks or adverse effects. Here are some guidelines for safe use of home remedies:

- **Research and understand the remedy:** Before using any home remedy, research it thoroughly to ensure you understand the ingredients, dosage, and potential side effects. Be cautious of any remedy that makes lofty or unrealistic claims.

- **Consult with your doctor:** If you have any underlying health conditions or are taking medications, it's always a good idea to consult with your doctor before trying any home remedies.

- **Follow instructions carefully:** Make sure to follow the instructions carefully and don't improvise or add extra ingredients to the recipe.

- **Be mindful of allergies:** If you have any known allergies to certain foods or ingredients, make sure to check that they're not present in the home remedy before using it.

- **Use high-quality ingredients:** Use only high-quality, fresh, and pure ingredients for your home remedies. Avoid using expired or contaminated products.

- **Start with small doses:** When trying a new remedy, start with a small dose to see how your body reacts. If there are no adverse effects, you can gradually increase the dosage as recommended.

- **Monitor for side effects:** Be vigilant for any adverse reactions or side effects, such as skin irritation, gastrointestinal upset, or allergic reactions.

- **Discontinue use if necessary:** If you experience any adverse effects or if the remedy is not working as intended, discontinue use and seek medical advice.

- **Keep it out of reach of children:** Store any home remedies out of reach of children to prevent accidental ingestion or misuse.

By following these guidelines, you can safely use home remedies to treat various ailments and improve your overall health and wellness.

possible side effects of home remedies

Home remedies can be a natural and cost-effective way to treat various health problems. However, they may also have side effects that people should be aware of. Some of the possible side effects of home remedies include:

- **Allergic reactions:** Some natural remedies may cause allergic reactions in certain individuals. For example, people who are allergic to certain herbs or plants may experience an allergic reaction if they consume or apply them.

- **Skin irritation:** Certain home remedies, such as lemon juice or vinegar, may cause skin irritation or even burns if applied in excessive amounts or without proper dilution.

- **Digestive issues:** Some natural remedies, such as ginger or garlic, may cause digestive issues like stomach upset, diarrhea, or bloating.

- **Interaction with medications:** Some home remedies may interact with certain medications, making them less effective or causing adverse effects. For example, taking large amounts of garlic may increase the risk of bleeding when taken with blood-thinning medications.

- **Overdose:** Some natural remedies can be toxic in large amounts. For instance, consuming too much licorice root can lead to high blood pressure, low potassium levels, and other serious health problems.

It is always essential to do thorough research before trying any home remedies and consult with a healthcare professional if you have any underlying medical conditions or are taking medications to avoid potential side effects.

When to seek medical attention over remedies

While home remedies can be helpful for minor ailments, there are certain situations when seeking medical attention is necessary. Here are some guidelines for when to seek medical attention:

- **Symptoms persist or worsen:** If your symptoms do not improve or worsen after a few days of trying home remedies, it may be time to see a doctor.

- **Severe pain:** If you experience severe pain that is not relieved by over-the-counter pain medications, you should seek medical attention.

- **Difficulty breathing:** If you are having difficulty breathing, seek medical attention immediately.

- **High fever:** If you have a fever of 103°F or higher, you should seek medical attention.

- **Persistent vomiting or diarrhea:** If you are experiencing persistent vomiting or diarrhea, especially if it is accompanied by dehydration or other symptoms, seek medical attention.

- **Head injury:** If you have experienced a head injury, seek medical attention immediately, especially if you experience symptoms such as confusion, dizziness, or loss of consciousness.

- **Chest pain:** If you experience chest pain, seek medical attention immediately.

- **Allergic reactions:** If you experience an allergic reaction, such as difficulty breathing or swelling of the face, seek medical attention immediately.

Remember, it's always better to err on the side of caution and seek medical attention if you are unsure about the severity of your symptoms.

Conclusion

Home remedies have been used for centuries to treat minor illnesses and alleviate symptoms. Many natural remedies have been found to have healing properties and can be used to supplement medical treatments. Some of the most commonly used home remedies include herbal teas, essential oils, hot compresses, honey, and ginger.

While home remedies may be effective in treating minor ailments such as headaches, sore throats, and stomach upsets, they should not be relied upon solely for the treatment of serious illnesses or medical conditions. It is always recommended to seek professional medical advice before trying any home remedy, especially if you have a chronic or serious medical condition, or are taking medication.

In conclusion, while some home remedies may provide relief for minor ailments, they should not replace professional medical advice or treatment. It is important to always consult with a healthcare professional before trying any home remedies or alternative treatments.

Recap of the benefits of using home remedies

Home remedies are natural and affordable treatments that can be used to address various health concerns. Here are some potential benefits of using home remedies:

- **Cost-effective:** Home remedies typically use ingredients that are easily accessible and affordable, making them a cost-effective alternative to prescription medications or over-the-counter treatments.
- **Natural:** Home remedies use natural ingredients, which can be gentler on the body and may have fewer side effects than synthetic or chemical-based treatments.
- **Customizable:** Home remedies can be customized to fit individual needs and preferences. For example, someone with sensitive skin may be able to adjust the ingredients in a facial mask recipe to avoid irritation.
- **Convenient:** Home remedies can often be made with ingredients that are already on hand in the kitchen or pantry, making them a convenient option for minor health concerns.
- **Sustainable:** Using home remedies can be a more sustainable choice than relying on packaged products, as it reduces the amount of waste generated by disposable packaging.

It is important to note that while home remedies can be effective for certain health concerns, they may not always be appropriate or safe for more serious or complex conditions. It is always best to consult with a healthcare professional before trying any new treatment, especially if you have a preexisting medical condition or are taking medication.

Encouragement to explore natural remedies as a complement to modern medicine.

Exploring natural remedies as a complement to modern medicine can be a great way to support your overall health and well-being. While modern medicine has many benefits, including advanced treatments and diagnostic tools, natural remedies can offer additional support and benefits that may not be found in pharmaceuticals.

Many natural remedies have been used for centuries to treat a variety of ailments and conditions. They are often derived from plants, herbs, and other natural sources, and can be used in a variety of ways, such as through teas, tinctures, oils, and supplements.

Natural remedies can offer a range of benefits, including reducing inflammation, boosting the immune system, promoting relaxation and reducing stress, improving digestion, and supporting overall health and well-being. They can also be a safer and more cost-effective alternative to prescription medications, which can come with a range of side effects.

It is important to note that natural remedies should not replace modern medicine, especially for serious or life-threatening conditions. However, they can be a valuable complement to modern medicine, helping to support your overall health and well-being.

If you are interested in exploring natural remedies, it is important to do your research and talk to a qualified healthcare professional, such as a naturopathic doctor or herbalist. They can help you understand which remedies may be most beneficial for your specific needs and health concerns, and can work with you to create a holistic and personalized health plan.